HEAVY TRUTH

Understanding Obesity in the Modern World

Dr. Bernd Kortig

TABLE OF CONTENTS

<u>TREATMENT AND MANAGEMENT OF OBESITY</u>

<u>PREVENTION OF OBESITY</u>

<u>CONCLUSION</u>

INTRODUCTION: UNDERSTANDING OBESITY

Obesity has become a global health epidemic, affecting millions of individuals across all age groups, socioeconomic backgrounds, and geographical regions. Defined as a condition characterized by excessive accumulation of body fat, obesity is not merely a cosmetic concern but a complex medical problem with far-reaching consequences. Understanding obesity requires exploring its multifaceted nature, encompassing biological, environmental, psychological, and societal factors.

Defining Obesity:

At its core, obesity is often defined by an excessive accumulation of body fat that presents a risk to health. The most common measure used to classify obesity is the Body Mass Index (BMI), which calculates an individual's body fat based on their height and weight. While BMI serves as a useful screening tool, it has limitations, such as not accounting for variations in body composition or distribution of fat. Other methods, such as waist circumference and waist-to-hip ratio, provide additional insights into the distribution of body fat and associated health risks.

Historical Context:
Obesity is not a new phenomenon; its roots can be traced back through human history. However, the prevalence of obesity has dramatically increased over the past few decades, leading to its classification as an epidemic. Historical factors, such as changes

in diet, lifestyle, and food production, have contributed to the rise in obesity rates. Moreover, societal shifts, including urbanization, technological advancements, and changes in employment patterns, have altered the way people live, work, and eat, further exacerbating the obesity crisis.

Prevalence and Trends:
The prevalence of obesity has reached alarming levels worldwide, affecting individuals of all ages and socioeconomic backgrounds. According to the World Health Organization (WHO), global obesity rates have nearly tripled since 1975, with more than 1.9 billion adults classified as overweight, of whom over 650 million are obese. Additionally, childhood obesity rates have soared, raising concerns about the long-term health implications for future generations. These trends underscore the urgent need for comprehensive strategies to

address and mitigate the impact of obesity on public health.

Biological Factors Contributing to Obesity: Obesity is influenced by a complex interplay of genetic, physiological, and metabolic factors. Genetic predisposition plays a significant role in determining an individual's susceptibility to obesity, with certain gene variants increasing the risk of weight gain and adiposity. Additionally, hormonal imbalances, such as leptin resistance and dysregulation of appetite-regulating hormones, can disrupt the body's energy balance and contribute to weight gain. Furthermore, metabolic factors, including insulin resistance and impaired lipid metabolism, can promote the development of obesity and related metabolic disorders.

Environmental and Lifestyle Influences:

Beyond genetics, environmental and lifestyle factors play a pivotal role in shaping obesity risk. The modern obesogenic environment is characterized by easy access to high-calorie, nutrient-poor foods, ubiquitous advertising of unhealthy products, and sedentary lifestyles. Food deserts, limited access to fresh and nutritious foods, and socioeconomic disparities exacerbate the problem, disproportionately affecting marginalized communities. Additionally, cultural norms, social influences, and marketing practices can perpetuate unhealthy eating habits and sedentary behaviors, further contributing to the obesity epidemic.

Psychological and Sociocultural Dimensions: Obesity is not solely a physiological phenomenon but also has psychological and sociocultural dimensions. Emotional factors, such as stress, depression, and anxiety, can trigger overeating or unhealthy coping mechanisms, leading to weight gain and obesity. Moreover, societal attitudes and stigmatization of obesity can have profound effects on individuals' self-esteem, body image, and mental well-being, perpetuating a cycle of weight gain and psychological distress. Addressing these psychosocial factors is essential for fostering a supportive and inclusive environment for individuals struggling with obesity.

THE SCIENCE BEHIND OBESITY

The science behind obesity is a multifaceted field encompassing a wide range of biological, physiological, genetic, and environmental factors that contribute to the development and progression of this complex condition. Understanding the intricate mechanisms underlying obesity is crucial for developing effective prevention and treatment strategies. In this section, we will explore the key scientific principles and concepts that shed light on the etiology and pathophysiology of obesity.

1. Energy Balance and Metabolism:
At its core, obesity results from an imbalance between energy intake and expenditure. The

body maintains its weight by balancing the calories consumed through food and beverages with the calories expended through basal metabolism, physical activity, and thermogenesis. When energy intake exceeds energy expenditure over an extended period, the surplus energy is stored as fat, leading to weight gain and eventually obesity. Conversely, when energy expenditure surpasses energy intake, the body draws upon its fat stores for fuel, resulting in weight loss.

2. Adipose Tissue Biology:
Adipose tissue, commonly known as fat, plays a central role in energy homeostasis and metabolic regulation. It is composed of adipocytes, specialized cells that store and release fat in response to energy demands. Adipose tissue is not merely an inert storage depot but an active endocrine organ that secretes various hormones, cytokines, and other signaling molecules collectively known

as adipokines. Dysregulation of adipokine secretion, particularly increased production of pro-inflammatory adipokines such as leptin and decreased production of anti-inflammatory adipokines such as adiponectin, is implicated in the pathogenesis of obesity-associated metabolic disorders.

3. Hormonal Regulation of Appetite and Satiation:

Appetite regulation is governed by a complex interplay of hormonal signals originating from the gastrointestinal tract, adipose tissue, and central nervous system. Key appetite-regulating hormones include ghrelin, leptin, insulin, peptide YY (PYY), and glucagon-like peptide-1 (GLP-1). Ghrelin, often referred to as the "hunger hormone," stimulates appetite and promotes food intake, whereas leptin, produced by adipose tissue, acts as a satiety signal, signaling the brain to reduce food intake and increase energy expenditure. Dysregulation of these hormonal signals can disrupt appetite control mechanisms, leading to overeating and weight gain.

4. Genetic and Epigenetic Influences: Genetic predisposition plays a significant role in determining an individual's susceptibility to obesity. Numerous genes have been implicated in the regulation of body weight, appetite, metabolism, and fat distribution. However, obesity is not solely determined by genetics; environmental factors, lifestyle behaviors, and epigenetic modifications also play critical roles in shaping obesity risk. Epigenetic mechanisms, such as DNA methylation, histone modification, and non-coding RNA regulation, can modulate gene expression patterns in response to environmental cues, including diet, physical activity, and stress, thereby influencing

susceptibility to obesity and related metabolic disorders.

5. Neurobiology of Food Reward and Hedonic Eating:
The brain plays a central role in regulating food intake and energy balance through complex neural circuits involving regions such as the hypothalamus, brainstem, and reward pathways. The reward system, which encompasses dopaminergic pathways in the brain, mediates the pleasurable sensations associated with food consumption and motivates food-seeking behavior. Hedonic eating, characterized by the consumption of palatable, high-calorie foods for pleasure rather than hunger, can override physiological satiety signals and contribute to overeating and weight gain. Understanding the neurobiological mechanisms underlying food reward and hedonic eating is essential for developing interventions to mitigate the

impact of obesogenic environments on eating behavior.

THE ROLE OF DIET IN OBESITY

The role of diet in obesity is undeniably significant, as dietary habits play a central role in energy intake and expenditure, body weight regulation, and overall metabolic health. While genetics, physical activity, and other factors also contribute to obesity, the quality and quantity of food consumed are primary determinants of energy balance and weight status. In this section, we will explore various aspects of diet and their impact on obesity.

1. Macronutrient Composition:
The macronutrient composition of the diet—comprising carbohydrates, fats, and proteins—plays a critical role in influencing

energy balance and metabolic regulation. Diets high in refined carbohydrates and added sugars, such as those found in sugary beverages, processed foods, and sweets, can contribute to excessive calorie consumption and weight gain. Conversely, diets rich in fiber, whole grains, lean proteins, and healthy fats tend to promote satiety, regulate blood sugar levels, and support weight management.

2. Energy Density:
The energy density of foods refers to the number of calories per unit of weight or volume. Foods with high energy density, such as fried foods, desserts, and fast food items, often pack a significant number of calories in small servings, making it easy to consume excess calories without feeling full. In contrast, low-energy-density foods, such as fruits, vegetables, and broth-based soups, provide fewer calories per gram and can help

increase satiety while reducing overall calorie intake, thereby supporting weight loss efforts.

3. Portion Sizes:
Portion sizes have expanded dramatically over the past few decades, contributing to overeating and weight gain. Larger portion sizes not only provide more calories but also influence perceptions of appropriate serving sizes, leading individuals to consume more food than necessary. The normalization of oversized portions in restaurants, fast-food establishments, and packaged foods has fueled the obesity epidemic by encouraging excessive calorie consumption and undermining efforts to control portion sizes and calorie intake.

4. Nutrient Quality:
Beyond calorie content, the nutrient quality of the diet is essential for promoting overall health and well-being. A diet rich in

nutrient-dense foods, such as fruits, vegetables, whole grains, lean proteins, and healthy fats, provides essential vitamins, minerals, antioxidants, and phytonutrients that support optimal metabolic function and reduce the risk of chronic diseases. Conversely, diets high in processed foods, refined carbohydrates, trans fats, and excessive sodium can contribute to inflammation, insulin resistance, and metabolic dysfunction, increasing the risk of obesity and related comorbidities.

5. Dietary Patterns:
Rather than focusing solely on individual nutrients or foods, researchers increasingly recognize the importance of dietary patterns in influencing health outcomes, including obesity. Several dietary patterns have been associated with a lower risk of obesity and chronic diseases, such as the Mediterranean diet, DASH (Dietary Approaches to Stop

Hypertension) diet, and plant-based diets. These dietary patterns emphasize whole, minimally processed foods, abundant fruits and vegetables, healthy fats, and lean proteins while limiting added sugars, refined grains, and processed meats.

6. Behavioral Factors:

In addition to the nutritional composition of the diet, various behavioral factors influence dietary choices and eating behaviors, which, in turn, impact weight status. Environmental cues, social influences, emotional eating, stress, boredom, and other psychological factors can trigger overeating, unhealthy food choices, and disordered eating patterns, contributing to weight gain and obesity. Developing mindful eating practices, addressing emotional triggers, and cultivating a supportive food environment are essential for promoting healthier dietary habits and sustainable weight management.

7. Role of Ultra-Processed Foods:
Ultra-processed foods, characterized by their high levels of additives, preservatives, refined sugars, unhealthy fats, and artificial ingredients, have become ubiquitous in modern diets. These foods are often engineered to be highly palatable, convenient, and inexpensive, but they typically lack essential nutrients and fiber found in whole, minimally processed foods. Consuming a diet high in ultra-processed foods has been linked to weight gain, obesity, metabolic syndrome, and an increased risk of chronic diseases, highlighting the importance of prioritizing whole, nutrient-dense foods in the diet.

PHYSICAL ACTIVITY AND SEDENTARY LIFESTYLE

Physical activity and sedentary lifestyle are two interconnected aspects of human behavior that have profound implications for overall health, including the prevention and management of obesity. While physical activity refers to any bodily movement produced by skeletal muscles that requires energy expenditure, a sedentary lifestyle is characterized by prolonged periods of sitting or low levels of physical activity. In this section, we will explore the importance of physical activity, the health risks associated with sedentary behavior, and strategies to promote a more active lifestyle.

1. Importance of Physical Activity:

Regular physical activity is essential for maintaining optimal health and well-being. Engaging in physical activity offers numerous benefits for both physical and mental health, including:

Weight management: Physical activity helps burn calories, build muscle mass, and increase metabolism, contributing to weight loss and weight maintenance.

Cardiovascular health: Exercise strengthens the heart, improves circulation, lowers blood pressure, and reduces the risk of heart disease, stroke, and other cardiovascular conditions.

Metabolic health: Physical activity improves insulin sensitivity, glucose regulation, lipid profiles, and overall metabolic function, reducing the risk of type 2 diabetes and metabolic syndrome.

Musculoskeletal health: Exercise strengthens bones, muscles, and joints, enhancing

mobility, flexibility, and balance, and reducing the risk of osteoporosis, osteoarthritis, and falls.
Mental well-being: Physical activity releases endorphins, neurotransmitters, and other chemicals that promote mood elevation, stress reduction, cognitive function, and mental resilience, lowering the risk of depression, anxiety, and other mental health disorders.

2. Health Risks of Sedentary Behavior: Prolonged sedentary behavior, such as sitting for extended periods, watching television, using electronic devices, and engaging in screen-based activities, has been associated with various adverse health outcomes, including:

Obesity: Sedentary behavior is a significant risk factor for weight gain and obesity, as it promotes energy imbalance and reduces calorie expenditure.

Cardiovascular disease: Sedentary behavior is linked to an increased risk of heart disease, stroke, and other cardiovascular conditions, independent of physical activity levels.

Type 2 diabetes: Sedentary behavior is associated with insulin resistance, impaired glucose metabolism, and an elevated risk of developing type 2 diabetes.

Metabolic syndrome: Sedentary behavior contributes to the clustering of metabolic risk factors, including abdominal obesity, hypertension, dyslipidemia, and insulin resistance, collectively known as metabolic syndrome.

Musculoskeletal problems: Prolonged sitting can lead to muscle stiffness, weakness, and imbalances, as well as back pain, neck pain, and other musculoskeletal issues.

Mental health disorders: Sedentary behavior is linked to an increased risk of depression, anxiety, stress, and other mental health disorders, as well as cognitive decline and dementia in older adults.

3. Strategies to Promote Physical Activity: Promoting physical activity requires a multifaceted approach that addresses individual, environmental, and societal factors. Some effective strategies include:

Individual interventions: Encouraging individuals to engage in regular physical activity by setting realistic goals, finding enjoyable activities, incorporating exercise into daily routines, and seeking social support from family, friends, or fitness groups. Environmental changes: Creating built environments that support active living, such as walkable neighborhoods, bike-friendly infrastructure, accessible parks, recreational facilities, and safe routes for walking and cycling.

Workplace initiatives: Implementing workplace wellness programs, standing desks, walking meetings, active breaks, and incentives to encourage employees to be more physically active during the workday.
School-based programs: Introducing physical education classes, recess breaks, extracurricular sports, active transportation initiatives, and healthy lifestyle education to promote physical activity among children and adolescents.
Policy measures: Implementing policies at the local, state, and national levels to promote physical activity, such as urban planning initiatives, transportation policies, land-use regulations, and funding for community programs and infrastructure improvements.

4. Reducing Sedentary Time:
In addition to promoting physical activity, reducing sedentary time is equally important for maintaining health and well-being. Some

strategies to reduce sedentary behavior include:

Taking frequent breaks from sitting: Breaking up prolonged periods of sitting with short bouts of standing, stretching, or light activity can help reduce sedentary time and improve circulation.

Incorporating movement into daily routines: Finding opportunities to stand, walk, or move throughout the day, such as taking the stairs, parking farther away, doing household chores, or gardening, can help offset sedentary behavior.

Limiting screen time: Setting limits on screen time for television, computers, smartphones, and other electronic devices, especially before bedtime, can help reduce sedentary behavior and promote better sleep hygiene.

Using activity trackers: Using wearable devices or smartphone apps to track daily steps, activity levels, and sedentary time can

raise awareness and motivate individuals to
be more physically active and less sedentary.

CHILDHOOD OBESITY

Childhood obesity is a significant public health concern characterized by excess body fat accumulation in children and adolescents. It is a complex and multifactorial condition influenced by a combination of genetic, environmental, behavioral, socioeconomic, and cultural factors. Childhood obesity poses immediate and long-term health risks, including an increased risk of chronic diseases, impaired physical and psychosocial development, and reduced quality of life. Understanding the causes, consequences, and prevention strategies for childhood obesity is essential for addressing this growing epidemic.

1. Prevalence and Trends:

The prevalence of childhood obesity has risen dramatically over the past few decades, reaching epidemic proportions worldwide. According to the World Health Organization (WHO), the number of overweight or obese children and adolescents aged 5-19 years has increased tenfold since 1975, with an estimated 38 million children under the age of 5 being overweight or obese in 2020. The prevalence of childhood obesity varies by region, country, socioeconomic status, and ethnic background, with higher rates observed in developed countries and urban areas.

2. Causes and Risk Factors:
Childhood obesity is influenced by a complex interplay of genetic, environmental, behavioral, and socioeconomic factors. Some common causes and risk factors include:

- Genetic predisposition: Children with a family history of obesity are at increased risk of developing obesity themselves, highlighting the role of genetic susceptibility.
- Environmental factors: The modern obesogenic environment, characterized by easy access to high-calorie, nutrient-poor foods, sedentary lifestyles, screen-based entertainment, and urbanization, promotes unhealthy eating habits and physical inactivity.
- Behavioral factors: Dietary behaviors, such as excessive consumption of sugary beverages, fast food, and processed snacks, as well as sedentary behaviors, such as prolonged screen time, lack of physical activity, and insufficient sleep, contribute to weight gain and obesity.
- Socioeconomic disparities: Children from low-income families and

marginalized communities are disproportionately affected by obesity due to limited access to healthy foods, recreational facilities, and healthcare services, as well as exposure to food insecurity, stress, and environmental toxins.

3. Health Consequences:
Childhood obesity is associated with a wide range of immediate and long-term health consequences, including:

- Metabolic disorders: Children with obesity are at increased risk of developing insulin resistance, type 2 diabetes, dyslipidemia, and metabolic syndrome, which can lead to cardiovascular disease and other chronic conditions later in life.
- Orthopedic problems: Excess weight places strain on the musculoskeletal

system, increasing the risk of joint pain, back pain, and orthopedic injuries, such as fractures and musculoskeletal deformities.

- Psychosocial issues: Children with obesity may experience stigma, discrimination, bullying, social isolation, low self-esteem, body dissatisfaction, depression, anxiety, and eating disorders, negatively impacting their mental health and quality of life.

- Developmental delays: Obesity can impair physical development, motor skills, cognitive function, academic performance, and social interactions, hindering children's overall development and educational attainment.

4. Prevention and Intervention:
Preventing and managing childhood obesity requires a comprehensive, multisectoral

approach that addresses the underlying determinants and risk factors while promoting healthy behaviors and environments. Some effective strategies include:

- Promoting breastfeeding: Breastfeeding provides optimal nutrition for infants and helps prevent childhood obesity by promoting healthy growth, appetite regulation, and metabolic health.
- Encouraging healthy eating habits: Providing children with a balanced diet rich in fruits, vegetables, whole grains, lean proteins, and healthy fats while limiting sugary beverages, fast food, processed snacks, and calorie-dense foods can help prevent obesity and promote overall health.
- Increasing physical activity: Encouraging children to engage in regular physical activity, active play,

sports, and recreational activities while minimizing sedentary behaviors, such as screen time and prolonged sitting, can support healthy growth, development, and weight management.

- Creating supportive environments: Schools, communities, healthcare settings, and policymakers can implement policies, programs, and initiatives that promote healthy eating, active living, and access to nutritious foods, safe recreational spaces, and healthcare services for children and families.

- Empowering families: Providing parents and caregivers with education, resources, skills, and support to make informed choices, role model healthy behaviors, and create a supportive home environment that fosters healthy eating, physical activity, and positive body image is essential for preventing childhood obesity.

PSYCHOLOGICAL FACTORS

Psychological factors play a crucial role in the development, maintenance, and management of obesity. Understanding the psychological dimensions of obesity is essential for addressing the complex interplay between thoughts, emotions, behaviors, and weight-related outcomes. In this section, we will explore various psychological factors associated with obesity, including emotional eating, stress, body image, self-esteem, and cognitive-behavioral influences.

1. Emotional Eating:
Emotional eating refers to the tendency to eat in response to emotional cues, such as stress, sadness, boredom, loneliness, or anxiety, rather than hunger or physical cues of hunger.

Many individuals use food as a coping mechanism to soothe negative emotions or alleviate psychological distress, leading to overeating, binge eating, and weight gain. Emotional eating can create a vicious cycle wherein negative emotions trigger overeating, followed by guilt, shame, and further emotional distress, perpetuating unhealthy eating patterns and weight-related struggles.

2. Stress and Coping Mechanisms:
Stress is a common trigger for emotional eating and weight gain. Chronic stress activates the body's stress response system, leading to the release of cortisol and other stress hormones, which can increase appetite, promote cravings for high-calorie foods, and contribute to abdominal fat accumulation. Moreover, stress can disrupt sleep, impair self-regulatory mechanisms, and undermine coping strategies, making it more challenging

to manage weight and adopt healthy lifestyle behaviors. Developing effective stress management techniques, such as mindfulness, relaxation techniques, social support, and cognitive-behavioral therapy, is essential for mitigating the impact of stress on eating behavior and weight management.

3. Body Image and Self-Esteem:
Body image refers to an individual's perceptions, thoughts, feelings, and attitudes towards their own body size, shape, and appearance. Poor body image and low self-esteem are common psychological factors associated with obesity and weight-related struggles. Societal pressures, cultural norms, media portrayals, and interpersonal experiences can contribute to distorted body image perceptions, negative self-talk, and self-criticism, fostering feelings of inadequacy, shame, and worthlessness. Moreover, weight stigma, discrimination, and

societal biases against larger bodies can further erode self-esteem and perpetuate negative body image beliefs, contributing to disordered eating behaviors and psychological distress.

4. Cognitive-Behavioral Influences: Cognitive-behavioral factors play a significant role in shaping eating behaviors, weight management efforts, and treatment outcomes for obesity. Cognitive distortions, such as all-or-nothing thinking, overgeneralization, and catastrophizing, can undermine self-efficacy, motivation, and adherence to healthy lifestyle changes. Moreover, maladaptive beliefs and attitudes about food, weight, and body shape, such as rigid diet rules, food labeling (e.g., "good" foods vs. "bad" foods), and weight-based self-worth, can perpetuate disordered eating patterns and hinder progress towards weight goals. Cognitive-behavioral therapy (CBT)

and other evidence-based interventions target these cognitive distortions and maladaptive beliefs, helping individuals develop healthier attitudes towards food, body image, and self-care.

5. Social Influences and Support:
Social factors, including family dynamics, peer relationships, cultural influences, and societal norms, shape eating behaviors, attitudes towards food, and weight-related perceptions. Family environment, parental modeling, and food-related practices can influence children's eating habits and weight trajectories from an early age. Moreover, social support from family, friends, healthcare providers, and support groups can play a vital role in promoting behavior change, providing encouragement, accountability, and practical assistance in adopting healthier lifestyle habits. Building a supportive social network and fostering

positive social connections can enhance resilience, motivation, and long-term success in weight management efforts.

TREATMENT AND MANAGEMENT OF OBESITY

Treatment and management of obesity involve a multifaceted approach that addresses various aspects of an individual's lifestyle, including diet, physical activity, behavior modification, and sometimes medical intervention.

Dietary Modifications:

- Caloric Restriction: Consuming fewer calories than the body expends is essential for weight loss. This can be achieved through portion control, reducing intake of high-calorie foods, and increasing consumption of fruits, vegetables, lean proteins, and whole grains.

- Nutritional Counseling: Working with a registered dietitian can provide personalized guidance on healthy eating habits and meal planning tailored to individual needs and preferences.
- Behavioral Strategies: Techniques such as mindful eating, keeping food journals, and setting realistic goals can help individuals make sustainable changes to their eating habits.

Physical Activity:

- Regular Exercise: Engaging in moderate-intensity aerobic activity, such as brisk walking, swimming, or cycling, for at least 150 minutes per week is recommended for weight management. Strength training exercises can also help build muscle mass and boost metabolism.

- Lifestyle Changes: Incorporating physical activity into daily routines, such as taking the stairs instead of the elevator or walking instead of driving for short distances, can contribute to overall calorie expenditure.

Behavioral Therapy:

- Cognitive-Behavioral Therapy (CBT): CBT techniques aim to identify and modify unhealthy thoughts and behaviors related to food, eating, and physical activity. This type of therapy can help individuals develop coping skills, manage stress, and address emotional triggers for overeating.
- Support Groups: Joining support groups or weight loss programs can provide accountability, encouragement,

and practical tips for overcoming obstacles to weight management.

Medical Intervention:

- Prescription Medications: Certain medications may be prescribed to aid weight loss by suppressing appetite, reducing fat absorption, or increasing feelings of fullness. These medications are typically recommended for individuals with a body mass index (BMI) of 30 or higher or those with a BMI of 27 or higher with obesity-related health conditions.
- Bariatric Surgery: In cases of severe obesity or when other weight loss methods have been ineffective, bariatric surgery may be considered. Procedures such as gastric bypass, gastric sleeve, or gastric banding can significantly reduce stomach capacity

and/or alter the digestive process to promote weight loss.
- Close Monitoring and Follow-up: Regular monitoring of weight, dietary habits, physical activity, and potential side effects of medications or surgical procedures is crucial for long-term success and maintenance of weight loss.

Psychological Support:

- Addressing Underlying Issues: Obesity can be influenced by psychological factors such as trauma, depression, anxiety, or low self-esteem. Seeking therapy or counseling to address these underlying issues can support weight management efforts.
- Body Image and Self-Esteem: Building a positive body image and self-esteem is essential for long-term success in

managing obesity. Practicing self-compassion, focusing on non-weight-related goals, and surrounding oneself with supportive individuals can help foster a healthy relationship with one's body.

Lifelong Maintenance:

- Continued Support: Successful weight management requires ongoing commitment and support. Regular check-ins with healthcare providers, participation in support groups or maintenance programs, and continued focus on healthy habits are essential for maintaining weight loss and preventing weight regain.
- Healthy Habits: Emphasizing sustainable lifestyle changes, rather than short-term diets or extreme measures, is key to maintaining

long-term weight loss. This includes prioritizing balanced nutrition, regular physical activity, adequate sleep, stress management, and self-care practices.

PREVENTION OF OBESITY

Preventing obesity involves a combination of individual lifestyle changes, community interventions, policy initiatives, and societal efforts to create environments that support healthy behaviors.

Promoting Healthy Eating Habits:

- Education and Awareness: Providing information on the importance of balanced nutrition, portion control, and the benefits of consuming fruits, vegetables, whole grains, lean proteins, and healthy fats can empower individuals to make healthier food choices.
- Access to Nutritious Foods: Ensuring access to affordable, fresh, and healthy

foods in all communities, including low-income neighborhoods and rural areas, can facilitate healthier eating habits.

- Nutrition Labeling: Clear and easy-to-understand nutrition labeling on food products can help consumers make informed choices about the foods they purchase and consume.

Encouraging Physical Activity:

- Physical Education in Schools: Incorporating regular physical education classes and opportunities for physical activity throughout the school day can help children develop healthy exercise habits from a young age.
- Active Transportation: Promoting walking, biking, or using public transportation can encourage

individuals to incorporate physical activity into their daily routines.

- Community Recreation Programs: Providing access to parks, recreational facilities, walking trails, and community sports leagues can make it easier for people of all ages to engage in physical activity.

- Workplace Wellness Programs: Employers can implement workplace wellness initiatives that encourage employees to be more active during the workday, such as walking meetings, onsite fitness classes, or incentives for using stairs instead of elevators.

Creating Supportive Environments:

- Healthy Food Environments: Implementing policies that promote healthier food options in schools, workplaces, restaurants, and other community settings can help individuals make better dietary choices.

- Physical Activity-Friendly Communities: Designing neighborhoods and urban environments that prioritize pedestrian safety, access to parks and recreational spaces, and infrastructure for walking and biking can encourage physical activity.

- Media and Marketing: Regulating advertising of unhealthy foods and beverages, particularly targeted at children, and promoting positive messages about nutrition and physical activity in media and marketing campaigns can help shape societal norms and behaviors.

Preventing Early Childhood Obesity:

- Prenatal and Early Childhood Nutrition: Providing education and support to pregnant women and new parents on the importance of breastfeeding, introduction of healthy solid foods, and promoting healthy growth and development can help prevent early childhood obesity.

- Early Childhood Education: Incorporating nutrition education and physical activity into early childhood education settings, such as preschools and daycare centers, can establish healthy habits that can last a lifetime.

Policy and Advocacy:

- Food and Beverage Policies: Implementing policies that restrict the marketing and availability of unhealthy foods and beverages in schools, childcare settings, and public spaces can create environments that support healthy choices.

- Urban Planning: Incorporating health considerations into urban planning and transportation policies, such as zoning regulations that encourage mixed-use developments, walkable neighborhoods, and access to green spaces, can promote physical activity and reduce obesity rates.
- Government Initiatives: Supporting government initiatives at the local, state, and national levels that promote healthy eating, active living, and obesity prevention through funding, research, and policy development can have a significant impact on population health.

Family and Social Support:

- Family Meals: Encouraging regular family meals and involving children in meal preparation can promote healthier eating habits and foster positive relationships with food.

- Social Support Networks: Building social support networks that promote healthy behaviors and provide encouragement, accountability, and resources for individuals and families striving to maintain a healthy weight can be instrumental in preventing obesity.

CONCLUSION

The journey through the complex landscape of obesity has illuminated the intertwined factors contributing to its rise and the multifaceted strategies essential for prevention and management. From exploring the physiological mechanisms underlying weight regulation to delving into the societal, environmental, and psychological influences shaping our behaviors, this book has sought to provide a comprehensive understanding of obesity.

We have witnessed the profound impact of lifestyle choices, socioeconomic disparities, cultural norms, and environmental cues on our dietary patterns, physical activity levels, and ultimately, our waistlines. Yet, amidst the daunting statistics and the pervasive challenges, there exists a glimmer of hope—a recognition that obesity is not an insurmountable fate, but a condition that can be prevented and managed with concerted efforts at individual, community, and societal levels.

As we navigate the complexities of obesity prevention and management, it becomes evident that there is no one-size-fits-all solution. Instead, it requires a holistic approach that addresses the root causes while promoting sustainable lifestyle changes, fostering supportive environments, and advocating for policy reforms. It calls for collaboration among individuals, healthcare professionals, policymakers, educators, and community leaders to create a culture of health where nutritious foods are accessible, physical activity is encouraged, and well-being is prioritized.

Furthermore, it is imperative to approach obesity with empathy and understanding, recognizing the myriad factors—biological, environmental, and psychosocial—that influence an individual's weight. By destigmatizing obesity and embracing a compassionate, person-centered approach to care, we can empower individuals to embark on their own unique journeys toward health and well-being.

In the face of the obesity epidemic, let us not succumb to despair, but rather, let us be inspired by the resilience of the human spirit and the potential for positive change. Together, let us strive for a future where obesity is no longer a barrier to living a fulfilling, vibrant life—a future where every individual has the opportunity to thrive, irrespective of their size or shape. It is through collective action, unwavering determination, and unwavering compassion that we can build a healthier, happier world for generations to come.

www.ingramcontent.com/pod-product-compliance
Lightning Source LLC
Chambersburg PA
CBHW051848250726
48659CB00006B/2089